Chronic Fatigue Syndrome Cure

From Fatigued To Fabulous

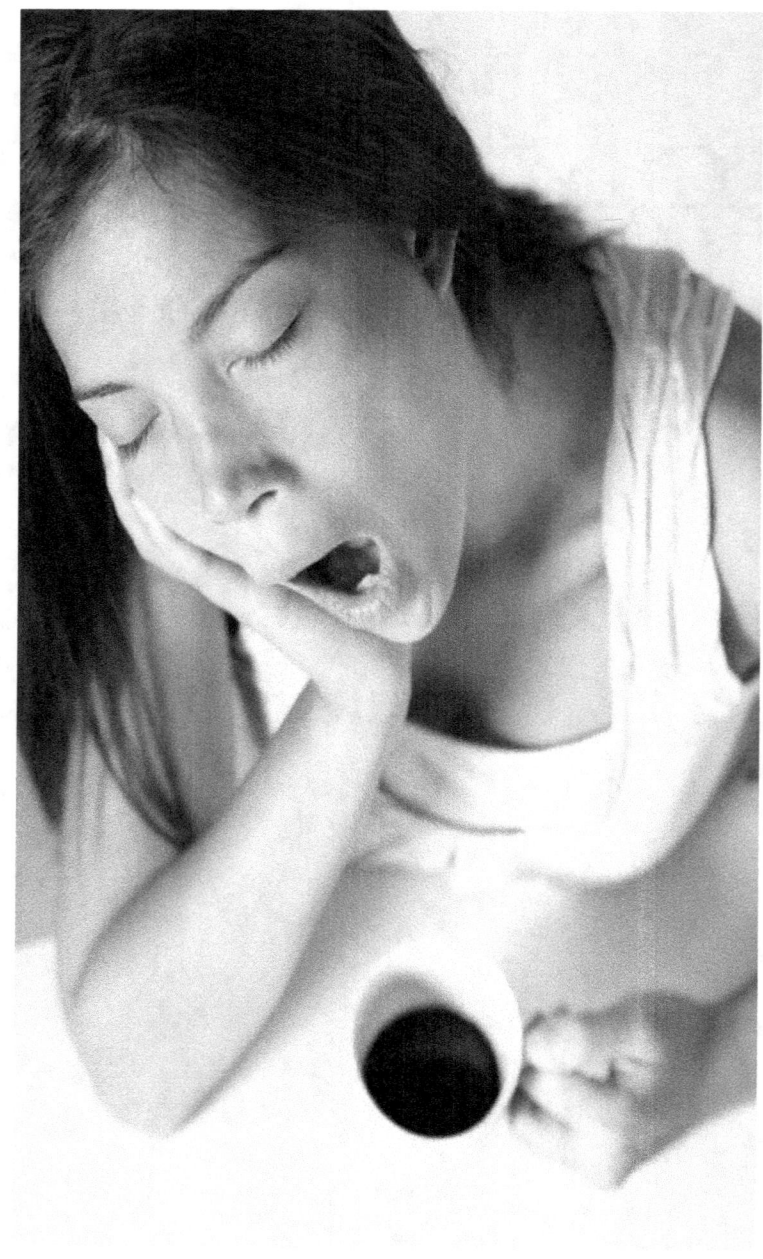

Chronic Fatigue Syndrome Cure

*From Fatigued To Fabulous
Stop Feeling Tired And Start
Living*

Rossie C Pattison

Rossie C Pattison

Copyright Notice

Contents

Preface: Chronic Fatigue Syndrome

Fatigue is more than merely "feeling tired." Chronic fatigue, as distinguished from the acute fatigue brought on by normal muscular activity, is actually an illness. And yet you may be fatigued to the point of physical collapse, and still not be fully aware of what is happening to you! Anyone who is tired because of strenuous or prolonged muscular activity ordinarily realizes his state of tiredness shortly after it begins to creep upon his body.

But chronic fatigue is so insidious a malady that frequently its very symptoms are an undue sense of restlessness and a need for excitement that spur the victim on to more and greater exhaustion. Sleep and relaxation have no great effect in re-living a fatigue that has gone far beyond these measures. Chronic fatigue can be fully overcome only by restoring to the body the nutritive elements whose absence caused the nerve breakdown in the first place.

The thousands upon thousands of chronic fatigue sufferers in this country today are unaware of their serious condition. And yet theirs are the abused, undernourished, starving nerve cells that mere rest will not benefit. Simple tiredness involves the muscles, whereas chronic fatigue involves the health of the nervous system and through it the health of the entire body.

Being tired in the simple, muscular sense of the word does not cause any change in the personality. But chronic fatigue, with all its dire implications, can change the disposition of the most even tempered person.

Before we can understand the seriousness of chronic fatigue, we must know something of the two nervous systems: the central nervous system and the sympathetic nervous system.

The sympathetic nervous system embraces all the nerve cells and fibers that supply the viscera, or vital internal organs: the lungs, heart, liver, kidneys, and intestines.

The central nervous system includes the spinal cord (nerve cable) and the brain. When the fetus is developing within the mother's uterus, the nerve tube folds up and its anterior end thickens to become the brain.

The central station of the nervous system is the medulla oblongata, which is the enlarged part of the spinal cord that forms the vital centers at the base of the brain. Here the respiration, muscle tension, blood pressure and other vital functions are controlled.

A broken neck is usually fatal because the break cuts off contact with these vital centers of the brain via the nerve cable in the spine. The central nervous system also controls all the sensory organs of the skin, as well as the skeletal muscles.

The nerve cells of which these two nervous systems are composed are called neurons. Millions of neurons make up a nerve fiber. These nerves, whether belonging to the sympathetic or the central nervous system, are as much an actual physical part of the body as the tongue or the bladder.

Like telephone wires, the nerves run throughout every part of the body, performing every function mental and physical, voluntary and involuntary.

The human body is nothing more than the sum and substance of its cells; and every one of the billions of cells is continuously active and in constant communication with the brain for months before the body emerges from the mother's womb, and up until the moment death silences the mind.

How is this constant communication between brain and body cells maintained? By the nerves of the central and sympathetic nervous systems, which in turn are made up of nerve cells, or neurons.

Every nerve cell has "temperament," the same as the human personality. A nerve cell possesses irritability, adaptability and conductivity. Each neuron acts like a runner in a relay race; the first cell in a nerve receives the impulse from the brain, explodes a charge of energy that passes the impulse on to the next cell, which sets off another charge of energy, and so on until contact is finally made with the muscle that is to be prodded into action.

Or this chain of reactions may move to the brain, as well as away from it, as happens when pain is felt in the finger and telegraphed to the brain. Nerve communication is a two way receiving and sending set receiving impulses from the brain and sending others back to the brain, incessantly, always working, even when the conscious mind is asleep.

The seat of all nervous energy is concentrated in the nerve cells, or neurons. Nerve cells must remain constantly charged with activity from long before birth up until the instant of death. These neurons are incessantly active; they need constant replenishment of their energy. Such replenishment of the nerve cells comes from relaxation and nutrition.

A nerve cell that is fatigued or famished is no longer adaptable, it is irritable, and its power of conductivity falls far short of normal. Of course the nerve cells do not maintain the same degree of activity at all times. The amount of energy they expend is governed by the demands put on them by the brain, that is, by you.

If a cell is made to expend its energy without a one hundred percent replacement of the energy used, it is like driving your car until five gallons of gas have been used, then driving into a filling station and having only four gallons put back into the tank. The day must eventually come when the gasoline tank is emptied!

And so it is with nerve cell energy. The neurons have a machine your body to keep operating in good condition. When they slow down, disease sets in; when they stop altogether, death takes place.

Nerve cell energy is required for as many "hidden" activities of the body as for those of which we are conscious. Breathing, digestion, glandular secretions, food assimilation, waste elimination all these are the "hidden" activities that make fully as many demands on the nerves as a game of tennis or a day's physical labor.

Nor is the activity of a nerve cell limited merely to giving out energy; the neuron must also work to take up energy. It is when the power of the nerve cell to take up energy is lessened that you become progressively more irritable, impulsive, and irresponsible and emotionally tense. And when this state of emotional upset progresses beyond a certain stage, the physical organs become affected. Chronic fatigue of mind and body has set in.

10

The reason for the instability of the emotions when nerve cell energy is at low ebb is because a nerve cell with depleted energy will explode more rapidly and more violently than is normally necessary when passing on an impulse to the next cell.

It is this heightened irritability of the nerve cell explosions that makes us aware of feeling "nervous" or "all in." Nature has set up a sort of "transformer" chain all along the lines of the two nervous systems to control the degree of consciousness with which the nerve impulses reach the brain. Every day we receive millions of impulses of which the conscious brain is barely aware, if at all.

Automatically these impulses are received in the brain, and then turned over to the subconscious mind to be acted upon. The reason why the conscious mind is kept from being swamped by awareness of these relatively unimportant impulses is because of the "transformer stations" set up all along the communication lines of the two nervous systems.

The purpose of these "transformer stations" is to control the intensity of the impulse flowing over the nerve wires, toning down the impulse to the desired volume by the time it reaches the brain. When the "transformer stations" are in good shape and working efficiently, the brain is protected from a flood of exaggerated impulses.

But when nerve exhaustion, resulting from inadequate relaxation and poor nutrition, throws these "transformer stations" out of good working order, the brain is harassed by a multitude of impulses that have no great consequence, yet each of which is clamoring for immediate and individual attention.

It is this jangling of uncontrolled nerve impulses, slipping past the broken-down "transformer stations" without being toned down, that brings on the physical and mental symptoms of chronic fatigue in its varying degrees.

The lower the nerve cell energy in these "transformer stations" along the nerve communication lines, the greater the flood of unwanted impulses that reaches the conscious brain, only to be transmitted right back to the physical organs in the form of uncontrolled emotional impulses.

Decreased energy in the nerve cells increases the volume of irritating impulses that reach the brain an undesirable volume that, sooner or later, will result in chronic fatigue.

You may have noticed that I keep designating it as "chronic" fatigue. This is done to impress more emphatically upon you the fact that there are forms of fatigue which no longer will respond to rest alone.

Neurologists divide the scale of nerve cell energy into six degrees, ranging from perfect health to death, with in-between degrees of neurasthenia, melancholia, mania and exhaustion.

When the body is healthy, when enough rest is being obtained and nutrition is good, the nerve cell energy is at par, and a sensation of wellbeing is experienced by mind and body.

But, as the energy in the nerve cells begins to drop lower and lower because of insufficient replacement (like the gasoline in the automobile tank that is never completely refilled), the sensation changes from that of well-being to heightened nervous and physical symptoms.

Most victims of chronic fatigue hover around the so-called neurasthenic level, with symptoms that include restlessness, irritability, morning tiredness followed by a pep-up later in the day, persistent headaches, heartburn, indigestion pains, constipation or diarrhea (or an alternating siege of both), vague fears and anxieties, and shooting pains throughout the body.

For individuals who have reached this stage of energy depletion in the nerve cells that this chapter is addressed. For it's you-- whose fatigue has become chronic to the danger point.

According to Sir James Paget, famous British physician: "You will find that fatigue has a larger share in the promotion and transmission of diseases than any other single causal condition you can name."

There is proof of Sir James' enlightening statement in the fact that nearly every disease, whether minor or serious, is characterized by the early symptoms of fatigue. And this brings up the old" which came first the chicken or-the egg" question: Does disease cause fatigue or does fatigue bring on disease?

Introduction

Physicians may go on for years treating patients for muscular ailments, heart disorders or disturbances of the gastro-intestinal tract, to say nothing of dozens of other maladies, and yet the patient often will show little or no improvement, despite the most intelligent medical treatment available. Why?

Because these illnesses are, in reality, nothing but symptoms of drastically low nerve cell energy! Far more improvement in the general symptoms of chronic fatigue is to be found in restoring the power of the nerve cells to take up energy than in giving doses to alleviate outward symptoms of inward exhaustion.

If you were to get a cinder in your eye, the logical action would be to remove the cinder first, then to apply soothing applications to the irritated eye. You would have little faith in the healing ability of anyone who would try to relieve the pain caused by a foreign object by merely placing hot applications to the eye. Your own common sense would tell you, "First get the cinder out, and then go about relieving the irritation."

That, exactly, is the way I feel about the average treatment given the victim of chronic fatigue. First get at the seat of the trouble; restore the power of the nerve cells to take on energy. Then go about treating the damage done to the physical organs by the chronically fatigued nervous system.

The day must come when psychiatry, medical research and nutritional therapy will blend the benefits of their specialized knowledge into one great healing profession one that will come to look upon man first as a mass of cells that are always hungry, never resting, highly susceptible to irritation and starvation.

Second, they will see man as a body animated and dominated by a combined nervous system that has to remain energized to the peak of its capacity to absorb energy from the bloodstream in the form of nutrients, if the body parts are not to be abused by an overwrought mind.

And third they will regard man as a set of physical organs, the disorders and diseases of which serve as indicators of his nerve cell energy. There is no way to measure nerve cell energy as one would register the heart beat or analyze the red blood cell count.

It is only when the mind, through the central and sympathetic nervous systems, has allowed the bodily organs to become ill that a clue is obtained as to the low level to which nerve cell energy has fallen.

Of course, when I say "bodily organs" that includes the brain too since it is a very vital physical organ. And when the cells of the brain, like those of the heart or the intestines, become affected by an exhausted nervous system, this mental organ develops very definite symptoms that take the form of irrational thinking, excitability, despondency and uncontrolled emotional impulses.

For that reason, we are likely to think of these as "mental" symptoms, whereas actually they are as physical as the pain that strikes the pit of the stomach. Please do not get the idea from any of the above that several nights of inadequate rest, or a few meals lacking in nutritional value are going to set you on the road to chronic fatigue.

Nature has taken care of our occasional lapses by setting up a reserve of nervous energy that will restore the neurons to maximum efficiency when their energy falls below the level at which body health is maintained.

It is only when we draw too heavily on this reserve of nervous energy without giving it; too, a chance to build up that the fat is in the fire! Chronic fatigue does not result as a consequence of two or three days' wrong living, or even a month or two: chronic fatigue comes from a long-term accumulation of bad eating and living habits.

There are several outstanding reasons why chronic fatigue has become almost a national malady, a sort of "American disease." Deliberate starvation, undertaken with the mistaken idea of losing weight by eating meals woefully inadequate in most nutritive elements, is a common reason for chronic fatigue.

From the lecture platforms, and in my previous books, I have implored my female listeners not to ruin their health in a mistaken pursuit of their figures.

While I agree that unnecessary fat is destructive to beauty and may be injurious to general health, I have seen what faulty reducing diets can do to otherwise normal, healthy bodies and nerves. And I urge all to undertake no reducing diet unless it contains all the necessary food elements minerals, vitamins and protein (amino acids).

If necessary, fortify yourself against undernourishment by adding dietary supplements in concentrated form, particularly the protein which every nervous system, every set of vigorous muscles and everybody-mass of living cells must have in bountiful supply to maintain mental and physical health.

A victim of chronic fatigue came to my attention recently. She recited a list of symptoms headaches, extreme weariness, digestive upsets, and despondency alternating with nervous exhilaration.

But it was not difficult to get at the root of this woman's case, for her very appearance provided the clue. Her muscles were flabby, the skin hung loosely on her face, throat and arms; she was pale and sunken-eyed. Deliberate starvation of the tissue and nerve cells had allowed her to gloat over a forty-pound weight loss in only eight weeks, but it had also brought on the chronic fatigue which she was now trying to overcome.

The quickest way I know of to commit nerve suicide is by prolonged, unsupervised dieting regimens that bring on chronic exhaustion of mind and body. Because toxins circulating in the bloodstream can poison body and nerve cells beyond their capacity to function properly, chronic constipation may also result in chronic fatigue.

Anyone living with a clogged intestinal tract is unfairly handicapping himself by harboring within his body toxic substances that sooner or later are bound to bring on chronic fatigue.

If the victims of prolonged constipation could be made to realize that the waste matter in their bowel is no less insidiously poisonous than the toxins produced by certain diseases, they might be goaded into giving more attention to this ailment that saps the body's energy by injuring the nerve cells.

Lack of enough vitamin B-1 (thiamin) is one of the most prevalent causes for chronic fatigue. Thiamin is the vitamin that specifically nourishes the nerve cells. For some time it has been recognized by the medical profession that liberal amounts of thiamin given to victims of nervous disorders will bring remarkable results.

And now, in the light of the more recent knowledge we have about the amazing power of thiamin and glutamic acid (one of the amino acids) to act upon the brain cells, it becomes increasingly evident that a serious lack of these two food elements can bring on chronic fatigue through malnutrition of the neurons of the central nervous system.

Undernourished nerve and brain cells are unequal to the hard work demanded of them every day by a body that must have sound thought and ready action in order to live fully.

Frequent spells of the "blues," irritability, mental and physical exhaustion can result from even a mild deficiency of thiamin in the diet. This fact, alone, is adequate proof of how vital this member of the B-complex group is to the health of mind and body.

Any diet, either reducing or normal, that does not include ample portions of beef and lamb (including the organs such as the liver, heart or kidneys) and whole grains is quite likely not to contain enough thiamin.

Pork, of course, is also high in thiamin, but I cannot recommend this meat. I have observed too many cases of digestive upsets resulting solely from eating pork, to say nothing of the serious disease, trichinosis, which comes, at times, from eating underdone pork.

Sometimes a diet that apparently should contain enough thiamin may be deficient enough in this "nerve vitamin" to bring on mild symptoms of chronic fatigue. This happens when a large percentage of the vitamin content is destroyed through improper handling and cooking.

Especially is this likely to happen to food prepared in restaurants where very little, if any, effort is made to serve meals that retain the fullest possible amount of vitamins and minerals.

Therefore, the only certain way to guard against the nerve starvation that brings on chronic fatigue is to supplement the diet with substantial doses of thiamin or a reliable vitamin B-complex, of which thiamin is a member.

Vitamin C also plays a part in controlling "brain fag" by contributing to the health of the blood vessels in the brain. This food element is often called the "capillary vitamin," for it contributes tone to the blood vessels of the body. In other words, vitamin C seems to "tighten" slackened blood vessels in the brain.

A blood vessel lacking in tone is too relaxed to allow normal circulation. When the blood vessels in the brain have lost their tone, naturally the brain cells are starving for the nutritive elements that, even though contained in the bloodstream, cannot be delivered quickly enough in large enough quantities to prevent "brain fag."

Therefore, in addition to thiamin and glutamic acid, the central nervous system, this includes the brain, needs vitamin C to assure healthy blood vessels and to keep circulation up to normal so that food elements in the blood may reach brain and nerve cells fast enough to restore lost energy.

Another dominant factor in nerve cell action is the mineral calcium. We shall see in a later chapter that a serious lack of calcium causes the sleep center of the brain to get out of order, resulting in insomnia.

Of the total quantity of calcium contained in the bloodstream, 99 per cent goes to the bones and teeth, with a small though very important 1 per cent being reserved for the blood, muscles and nerves. However, when the intake of calcium falls far below normal, it is quite likely that the bones and teeth take more than their share, leaving precious little calcium to fortify the nerve and muscle cells against fatigue.

To assure a proper balance in the body's utilization of calcium, it is safest to make certain that this very essential mineral is amply contained in the diet. Milk, of course, is one of the richest sources of calcium. But, unfortunately, many individuals cannot tolerate cow's milk because the curds it forms in the human stomach are often hard to digest.

Goat's milk is far easier to digest and contains equally high calcium content. But if goat's milk is not readily available, then calcium in tablet form is an excellent way of supplementing the diet with this mineral.

However, I must caution against using a tablet containing calcium in isolated form, since calcium should always be combined with sodium to keep it from depositing in the joints.

Sodium acts as the watchman to keep calcium properly distributed in the body. Even those persons who are able to drink liberal quantities of either cow's or goat's milk should make certain to eat liberally of the sodium foods such as celery, cucumbers, citrus fruits, lettuce, asparagus, etc.

The people of former centuries, and even those in the early decades of this century, did not suffer as widely from chronic fatigue as we do today. Their diets were not limited as narrowly as ours to artificial foods, and to foods grown on depleted soils, to say nothing of those fruits and vegetables most of whose vitamin value has been lost by being picked green and then being left in storage or in markets for days, even months, before reaching the table.

Chapter 1

Minerals and Vitamins

The serious lack of food-contained minerals and vitamins that the eating habits of this mid-twentieth century have brought into almost every home is helping promote the prevalence of chronic fatigue, our "American malady."

Then, when we stop to consider that bodies with seriously handicapped nerve and brain cells are trying to keep up the pace in our highly accelerated way of living, no wonder we find wrecked health, tortured nerves, and panicked minds on every hand. In fact, so much so that a whole new branch of healing psychiatry came into being to treat the poorly equipped minds and nerves trying to operate rundown bodies.

In other words, too many of us are trying to run the twentieth century race with a broken down model of a body. This can lead only to nervous disaster, as attested by the greatly increasing prevalence of chronic fatigue.

If habitual users of alcohol could see what they are doing to their nerve cells aside from any purely moral side of the question they might take heed of the warning to go slow with their drinking. Alcohol seriously depletes the body's reserve of vitamin B-complex.

Even though heavy users of alcohol were to eat well-balanced meals which they seldom do the high percentage of alcohol in the blood would absorb the vitamin B-complex, particularly the thiamin, preventing its reaching the nerve and body cells.

I do not intend to preach a temperance sermon: but, for your health's sake, if you must use alcohol, then be sure to add heavy amounts of vitamin B-complex in concentrated form to the diet.

While this measure will not cure your drinking habit only your own will power can do that it will help keep you off the alcoholic rocks of serious brain and nerve fatigue.

No one should be always tired! Any fatigue that lasts beyond the time it takes for normal rest to conquer normal tiredness is likely to have its origin in the nerves rather than in the muscles.

25

Nerve cells that are healthy can meet any circumstances without flinching, can perform any reasonable exertion without overburdening the muscles, and can maintain a normal balance between tiredness and relaxation.

But nerve cells starved for thiamin and calcium spurred on by brain cells undernourished for lack of glutamic acid and thiamine can lead to the destructive thinking and nerve exhaustion which usually results in the physical ailments known as mind-induced diseases.

The sensible way either to prevent the onset of chronic fatigue, or to help overcome the damage it has already done to mind and body, is to build nerve cell energy through reasonable periods of rest and relaxation and through protective nutrition. Nerve and brain cells steadied by the energy that comes from proper nourishment are the best defense against tense minds and chronic fatigue.

Chapter 2

Mind Caused Diseases

One of the difficulties about mind caused diseases is that they can imitate organic degeneration so closely it is often difficult to differentiate them from the real thing. The causes for these psychosomatic outbreaks are legion. Every case seems to stand alone in its true origin.

Take the case of Mary H.—pain for pain, Mary's illness could be matched by the symptoms of hundreds of other patients. Yet her complaint failed to respond to the ordinary treatments. Mary was the victim of an ailment brought on by an overwrought mind. But only after Mary had lost her appendix, her gall bladder, a section of intestine and one ovary did anyone suspect that perhaps Mary's trouble lay in her mind rather than in her abdomen.

27

Mary had been an extremely handsome woman, married to an adoring husband. The marriage was childless and all of her husband's devotion was centered on her. Back in the "depression thirties" Henry lost his hardware business and had to take a position as traveling salesman for a large concern.

His territory was far enough away to necessitate his being gone from home and Mary for as long as two and three months at a time. This was a difficult adjustment to make, especially since Mary and Henry had never been separated for more than a few days at a time in all the ten years of their marriage.

At first everything went along as ever. But then came the day when Henry, upon returning from a long absence, said to Mary, "Gosh, Baby, you're getting gray!"

As though that were not enough, he added fuel to the fire by remarking later on, "Gee, Honey, you better do something about those wrinkles in your neck. I don't want my wife to get old."

Because of these thoughtless remarks, Mary began to suspect that her husband no longer loved her, that while away from home he had met someone as beautiful as he once had thought her. She accused him of infidelity.

Henry was indignant and rushed out of the house. Mary suffered an acute attack of what her doctor called "appendicitis" and she was rushed to the hospital where she parted company with her appendix. Henry, contrite at this unexpected turn of events, returned and was duly forgiven.

But the seed of suspicion had been planted in Mary's mind, and she never let Henry forget that he was on probation. After a while, wearying of tearful accusations and vehement denials, he took up headquarters in a town within his territory. Mary remained at home, alone.

A divorce followed as a natural consequence of the estrangement likewise three more operations for Mary. The emotional strain had been too great for her gastro-intestinal tract; it retaliated in violent fashion.

There is no doubt that Mary was the victim of a mind-caused illness; that her agitated emotions had kicked up all the trouble in the first place, rather than her appendix.

But one question yet remains to be answered: Would Mary's mind have fallen under the domination of tense emotions if she had not first almost wrecked her nervous system by years of self-imposed starvation "dieting" she called it? Was not the underlying cause of her emotional breakdown to be found in the habitual malnutrition to which she had subjected her body for long intervals with the idea of retaining its "streamlines"?

If her entire physical machine had not been allowed to run down because of inadequate fuelling, would an emotionally upset mind have been able to stir up all that trouble in her abdomen?

These are questions the healing profession has yet to answer. These are questions on which I hope to throw some light in the succeeding chapters of this book.

The question arises: How can the mind make the body suffer ailments and diseases so apparently real that they defy detection from genuine organic breakdowns?

Before attempting to answer this question, I must ask another: Why should we treat mind and body as though they were two distinct, separate mechanisms? Isn't it wrong to speak of mind and body; shouldn't we learn, instead, to think in terms of mind-body?

The surface of a quiet pool is by no means separated from the bottom. A pebble dropped on the surface of that pool causes what appear to be surface ripples only; yet every atom of water in that entire pool is affected to some degree by this one action.

And so it is with the mind-body. What disturbs the brain waves will ultimately be reflected in the nerves, muscles and organs of the body. Sometimes the reaction is mild and fleeting, leaving no noticeable after-effects; but sometimes the reaction is so continual or so violent that it causes a general disturbance of body metabolism, with the result that pain and suffering are felt.

That valuable aid to criminal prosecution, the lie detector, is based on nothing more mysterious than the principle that what occurs in the mind will inevitably, and almost instantly, be reflected outwardly through certain changes in bodily functioning.

The suspect is asked a question deliberately calculated to induce fear or some other equally strong emotion. If he is innocent, there is no recorded physical reaction, simply because his mind does not harbor the emotional tensions that can produce these certain known bodily reactions.

On the other hand, if he is guilty, no human power can prevent the mind from entertaining thoughts of fear, anger or hatred as soon as certain questions are asked of the suspect. Instantly the by-products of these violent emotions become evident in the body; his pulse rate reflects a disturbed heartbeat. This is recorded on a chart by a supersensitive needle.

Therefore, even though the suspect may refuse to utter a word, his own thoughts will give him away! The reason for this is that the power exercised by the mind over our body, down to the last cell, is so great that every thought leaves its mark good, bad or indifferent upon the physical man.

So inseparable are brain waves from nervous, muscular and organic functioning that every thought is reflected involuntarily in some physical reaction. The theory of the lie detector is not entirely a modern one. In ancient days, when a crime had been committed, all suspects were rounded up and made to sit in a row on a bench. Each suspect was given a handful of uncooked rice to chew.

Why? Because the man guilty of the crime would have so dry a throat, owing to his fear of being found out, that he could not possibly chew and swallow dry rice with the same ease as the innocent man whose salivary glands were unaffected by fear.

Every human thought is recorded in some physical consequence. The body is like a sheet of paper upon which the mind writes.

For instance, there is the old parlor game of "mental telepathy." One person leaves the room, while those remaining decide upon an object the absent member is to guess, presumably from the strong thought waves projected into his mind by the intense concentration of those who know what the chosen object is.

Actually what happens is that one of the players "tells" the subject when he has guessed the correct object. Here is how it works: When the subject returns to the room, one of the persons who know the answer takes him by the hand.

As the subject wanders first to one side of the room, then to the other, unconsciously his "contact man" gives him signals through involuntary tugs of the hand whenever he strays in the wrong direction.

And when, by the process of elimination, the subject finally names the chosen object, he feels a quick, involuntary movement of the other person's hand. In other words, a muscular reaction caused by the emotion of surprise or approval registered in the mind of the person acting as guide. Now, a fleeting thought of disapproval, dislike, anxiety or fear may not make any serious, lasting impression upon the physical organs.

But when thoughts are permitted sometimes even encouraged by an underpar mind to form a regular bombardment of negative impressions, day in day out, year in year out, the vital bodily functions are bound to become affected.

A powerful hormone called adrenalin is secreted by the adrenal glands as a consequence of intense emotions; it is a secretion intended to carry the body through an emergency. But, like all emergency measures, it is too violent for constant use.

Therefore, the presence of adrenalin in the bloodstream when it is not needed is bound to exert too powerful an influence upon certain organs over too long a period. That, in brief, is the physiological basis for the harm done to the body by a tense mind.

Perhaps the harm may start with that first transient thought: "Wonder if I'll ever be a success?" An innocent enough thought; certainly no harm in it. But the thought pattern for this doubt has now been established. The next time it repeats itself; it becomes a little stronger, verging on the intensity of a minor fear: "Will I always be tied to this job I hate so much?"

And now the truly harmful mind-body cycle is on the verge of forming: Dissatisfaction, plus negative thinking, producing a total of fear and frustration which, in turn, will yield some undesirable physical consequences; perhaps digestive upsets, colitis, ulcers, high blood pressure, heart disorders even diabetes or tooth decay!

I wager that I can walk into a group of heart patients, or asthma sufferers, or arthritis victims and make a thought analysis that would strike home with more than one of those present. My "mind reading" would go something like this: There is someone here, I would say, who at some time in the past has entertained the thought: "Wonder if I'll ever get the breaks?" Next came the idea: "You have to have pulled to get along.

A little guy like me is lost in the shuffle." Soon this was followed by self-pity: "The boss doesn't recognize my true worth. He's got it in for me." Finally this dominant thought theme was established: "I'll never get anywhere. Everyone's against me. What's the use of trying?"

Perhaps it has been so long since these thoughts were conscious thinking that the patient, at first, could truthfully disclaim any memory of them. But let him bring the subconscious mind into play, and that miraculous storehouse of all thinking good and bad would soon drag forth remembrance of such thought patterns.

We cannot get very far in understanding how the mind can cause organic illness until we introduce this subconscious mind. We might try to explain it, in simple terms, as far as our present knowledge of it extends, by saying that the subconscious mind is the involuntary "recording machine and record player" of the conscious mind.

I have stressed the idea of "involuntary" because there is absolutely nothing voluntary or controllable about the subconscious mind. We exercise no control over our subconscious thinking. We can control our conscious mind, but our subconscious mind is no more controllable than the wind.

Chapter 3

The Subconscious Mind

The tone of our subconscious thoughts depends upon the general tenor of our conscious thinking. A morbid conscious mind is certain to produce morbid subconscious thoughts. Perhaps I should say that we cannot exercise direct control over our subconscious thoughts. Yet we can maintain a sort of indirect control over our subconscious mind by patrolling our conscious mind.

The subconscious mind records and stores every single thought or impression that is allowed to enter the conscious mind. If a Healthy, well-nourished brain permits only sane, positive thoughts to predominate in the conscious mind, and then the subconscious mind can record only sane, positive thinking.

The subconscious mind cannot invent ideas; this is a power given to the conscious mind alone. The singer who stands before the microphone can sing any combination of notes he desires; but the recording of that performance can do nothing more than to reproduce over and over again the original notes sung. And so it is with the subconscious mind; it can record and replay only the thoughts or thought combinations it has received from the conscious mind.

Nor are we able to say to the subconscious mind: "Stop sending those harmful thought impulses throughout my body!" All we can do is to weaken the undesirable thought recordings by causing the subconscious mind to record and broadcast the strong, insistent, positive thought impulses which a healthy conscious mind can be made to produce.

In other words, if the jangling, inharmonious thought recordings of the subconscious mind are undesirable, why not drown them out by louder and more frequent recordings of soothing, harmonious, productive thinking, deliberately provided by a healthy, well-controlled mind?

The theory of psychosomatic medicine is not entirely an original concept of this mid-twentieth century. Like many other healing methods such as the use of herbs and other natural substances the idea of healing the body through the mind is as old as the first witch doctor.

About all the witch doctor's mumbo-jumbo amounted to was an attempt at controlling the emotions of the afflicted one. In other words, the witch doctor was an aboriginal edition of a psychiatrist.

His psychological approach, strongly bolstered by his knowledge of herbs, often enabled the primitive witch doctor to effect cures which still puzzle modern medicine. A question arises at this point: Why, then, if the mind can cause illness, isn't everyone sick and afflicted, for goodness only knows we all have our share of worries and personal fears?

The answer to this is that not everyone worries and fears to the same degree. To some persons the fear of death, for instance, may be a faint buzzing in the mind, while to others it may roar like a tornado.

Naturally, those who "hear" this fear of death to such an extreme degree are those whose subconscious minds are going to record an exaggerated version of this fear, and whose bodies are going to react more violently to these emotional thought recordings.

One woman may feel a mild dislike for her mother-in-law; another woman, under almost identical circumstances, will despise her mother-in-law so intensely that her thought-action sequence is discolored by this hatred. One man may dislike being a bookkeeper, let us say, yet he does not let this dislike degenerate into self-pity. Instead, he turns his discontent into constructive action; he studies and applies himself so consistently that he is soon able to step into a position he does like.

On the other hand, the man most certain to become the victim of some mind-induced disease will go on as a bookkeeper, year after year, hating himself for not progressing, blaming those dependent upon him for "chaining" him to so antipathetic a job, despising those under whose supervision he must work for not recognizing he is capable of bigger things and yet never doing anything on his own to remedy a disagreeable situation!

What is the basic difference between the two women who dislike their mother-in-law, and between the two men who want to be something more important than a bookkeeper? In other words, what is the difference between those whose worries and fears roll off them like water off a duck's back, and those whose emotional reactions seem to permeate their innermost physical functioning?

Psychologists and psychiatrists, by way of explanation, would talk about "adjustments," "inhibitions," "thought processes," "reflexes," and so on. And, in the jargon of their professions, they would make sense.

But to the average man and woman such explanations are often more confusing and more fear-inducing than they are helpful. In as simple a way as I can with so complex a subject, I shall endeavor to offer my theory for the difference in emotional thought-control between the two wives, and between the two bookkeepers.

No one needs too much explanation of the physiological truth that a stomach constantly harassed with inferior, inadequate, in-digestible meals is the stomach most likely to become what is known as a "touchy" stomach.

Why, then, does not this same truth hold good for the brain, since it, too, is an organ of the body as surely as the stomach? A brain that is constantly abused, misused and undernourished develops into a "touchy" mind.

In other words, a mind that cannot winnow the chaff from the wheat in sane and harmful thinking; a mind that gradually loses voluntary domination over its thought patterns, surrendering its independence to the tyranny of wrong thinking; a mind that produces "nerves"; a mind that contributes to oversensitivity.

The person most likely to have his "feelings hurt" at the least offense is the one most disposed toward "irritable stomach," or colitis, or deafness, or asthma, and so on through the list of mind induced ailments.

It is difficult to fathom exactly where such a person's "irritable stomach" or "irritable bowel" ends and where his "irritable mind" begins. A personal slight, either real or fancied, is enough to send him off into an attack of indigestion or colitis. Perhaps a friend, acquaintance or fellow worker has merely made the general observation that "nobody is honest anymore."

Instantly, our sensitive person takes the remark as a slur on his personal honesty; he is offended; he broods on what has been said; he begins to dislike the person who made the remark; he may even fear that some little incident in his past (and most of us have such incidents in our pasts) has prompted this observation.

Yes, of course, it was aimed directly at him, no doubt about it. Now comes the stomach-ache or the colitis!

Or perhaps it was a clerk in a store who was rude. Immediately our sensitive person may bristle inwardly at the affront to his dignity as a customer, as an important person. And from that moment on his day is likely to produce some physical upset, all the way from a headache to a heart attack. I shall venture still further in my prognosis and say that the chances are nine out of ten that our sensitive, "irritable" person is also a person suffering from chronic fatigue.

Chapter 4

Fatigue and the Mental Health

Fatigue can be the result of mind-induced diseases or fatigue can cause the mental condition that paves the way for the onset of these same diseases. Fatigue, in other words, is a stealthy fellow who operates toward any goal, so long as that goal is an undesirable one!

Dr. Cowles in his excellent book entitled Don't Be Afraid proves that fatigue (or low nerve-cell energy, as he designates it) must first be allowed to attack the body before the mind can fall a ready victim to the onslaught of unreasonable fears or emotions.
And when fatigue has completely fastened itself upon the physical man, his weakened reasoning powers are all set to bring down upon his body any one or more of a host of painful, incapacitating illnesses.

42

Nor are these diseases easily distinguished from those resulting from genuine organic causes. A case of mind-induced colitis is as painful and as disabling as that resulting from actual damage to the colon.

I like the way Cowles draws a parallel between the human nervous system and a river dam. He says that little "dams" are set up all along the human nervous system, with one great "dam" in the brain, to hold back and keep in check the flood of nerve and thought impulses that would otherwise rush in upon our consciousness.

The lower a river dam is placed, the more water rushes over it. In exactly the same way, says Dr. Cowles, the lower the energy in our nerve cells, the greater the flood of impulses wanted or unwanted that beats against the brain.

Hence, the less energy there is in a nerve cell, the greater the irritability of that cell. A fatigued brain and nervous system that is, one made up of cells containing low nerve energy is inevitably an irritated brain. The brain, as an organ of the body the same as the liver, or the lungs, or the spleen is interlaced with infinitesimal, thread-like nerves.

Therefore, the brain in a tired, undernourished, ill-cared-for body is most assuredly going to be the brain with the greatest amount of irritability, and with the least ability to stabilize emotionally stimulated thought impulses by a reserve of reasoning power.

43

The young student who is found hanged, having taken his own life rather than face the disgrace of failure in his examinations, is more often than not the victim of an underpar brain where emotions were allowed to run away with reason.

A little more attention paid to the diet of our young people, with more insistence on plenty of rest and sane recreation, would save the lives of these unfortunate victims of overwrought, adolescent minds.

My belief is that no mental conflict strong enough to cause bodily illness or to engender the idea of suicide ever arose until the brain cells (because of general bodily malnutrition and fatigue) were so undernourished and so fatigued that the nerve cell energy reached a dangerously low ebb.

This belief is borne out by a recent experiment with a group of women whose diets were deliberately made almost free of thiamine, the "nerve" vitamin.

After a few weeks of this thiamine-deficient diet, two of the women became so depressed they had to be restrained from committing suicide! But when thiamine in adequate amounts was restored to the diet, their mental condition returned to normal.

This experiment, coupled with my own observations throughout years of work in nutritional therapy, prompts me to the theory that psychosomatic medicine must have its true basis in proper nutrition for the brain and nerve cells.

When the mind becomes undernourished and low in nerve cell energy, the slightest unpleasant or disturbing incident is projected by the conscious thinking into the subconscious mind, as though through a powerful magnifying glass.

What ordinarily would be of small or no consequence assumes the proportions of a major event when the mind is so underpar that it loses its sense of values.

Chapter 5

Fatigue Syndrome

A thirty-year-old mother had nursed her three young children through concurrent sieges of measles and whooping cough. No sooner were all the children off the sick list than her husband contracted double pneumonia and she remained at his bedside, taking only quick snatches of rest, until he had passed the crisis and begun to convalesce.

Not long after he had recovered sufficiently to return to work, the woman had to go on a long-delayed shopping tour for children's clothes. She went from one store to the next, seeking bargains, struggling through the crowds, getting more and more fatigued. Suddenly, upon entering the elevator of a large department store, her heart began to palpitate violently, her legs became too weak to support her, and a terrifying sensation of dying gripped her. She was taken home in an ambulance.

After a few days in bed, she was able to perform light household tasks. But she was afraid to venture again into public places, for fear of suffering another "heart attack." For years, although a young woman, she has remained cloistered in her home, living under the false idea of being a "heart" victim.

Actually what attacked this woman was an acute siege of fatigue. She was too run-down because of weeks of poor nutrition and in-adequate rest to have attempted an all-day shopping trip.

Yet, because her undernourished brain cells were too fatigued to reason the matter out for her, she grew to associate the horrible feeling of that "heart attack" with a public place. Thus her fatigue spawned a fear of going out in public. And, even more serious, her underpar mind sent enough fear thoughts to her heart to cause that organ to keep on acting as though it suffered from a real degenerative condition.

We must recognize that harmful thought patterns fear, hatred, anxiety, oversensitivity have their true origin in brain cell starvation and bodily fatigue. Such fatigue, which always has its origin in low nerve cell energy, is augmented by overwork, insufficient rest, continued emotional strain, inability to relax, intemperance and bad living habits, to name but a few of the most common fatigue "accomplices."

Summing it all up, we find the tendency toward poor thought habits has its initial cause in poor physical hygiene. That is why I stated earlier that it is difficult, even impossible, to draw a line and say conclusively that Mr. X's "nervous heart" is caused solely by his dissatisfaction with his job, or that Mrs. Y's colitis is caused exclusively by the resentment she feels toward her mother-in-law.

For, if Mr. X were not continuously run-down and irritable as a result of poor nutrition, he would probably look upon his job in a different light either as a stepping stone to something better, or as a blessing in disguise in a commercial world where depressions and unemployment may make any job a treasure to cherish.

If Mr. X were to pay more attention to the physical side of his welfare proper diet, more sleep, adequate recreation he might soon find his dissatisfaction tapering off. And just as certainly he would alleviate the symptoms of his so-called "nervous heart."

If Mrs. Y had not almost wrecked her digestive and nervous system by that strenuous "reducing diet" to the point where she drags through every day in a haze of fatigue sensations, she would very likely overlook the eccentricities of her mother-in-law as something to be endured for the sake of her husband's love.

But poor Mrs. Y is so fatigued, so underpar in every way because of malnutrition that whenever her mother-in-law comes to visit and is caught running her finger over the dust on the woodwork, Mrs. Y takes to her bed with a painful attack of colitis!

Do you see the point I am trying to make? So interrelated are the causes and effects of poor thinking, poor nutrition, poor hygiene and poor health that to try to single out the actual starting-point in the maze of mind-body ailments is like trying to find the end of the yarn in a tangled skein.

Chapter 6

Secret to Combat Mind-Induced Diseases

As a first and highly vital step, I advocate the building of as efficient a physical machine as possible, governed by a mind whose brain cells are tended and nourished as carefully as any expensive motor powering a high-priced piece of machinery. It is all very well for a patient to be told by a psychoanalyst that his fear of the dark stems from some childhood scare, and that his allergy results from this fear.

Yet if that patient's brain is not going to be strengthened and fortified to the maximum by means of proper physical measures, how can his allergy be overcome by making him realize that such a fear is ridiculous in an adult? Will the mind that was underpar enough to give sanctuary to such an unreasonable fear in the first place be strong enough to cast out that fear merely because it has been traced back to an early cause? Psychologists may have him repeat: "I'm not afraid in the dark; the dark is my friend; nothing can harm me."

But until that patient's underpar, physical organ called the brain is treated in the same efficient therapeutic manner in which a weakened heart or lung or kidney is treated that is, by proper restoration and fortification of the cells through correct feeding and elimination of wastes that brain is going to continue housing a mind beset by fancies, phobias and fears!

And these fancies, phobias and fears, if allowed to persist for any length of time to an intensified degree, are going to end up by breaking out in the form of one or more of the psychosomatic ailments already mentioned. What we must realize, if we are not to become a race of misfits and semi-invalids in this Early Atomic Age, is that unnatural (some call it "civilized") living brings on fatigue.

Fatigue lays the groundwork and unreasoning fears and uncontrollable emotions.
And these harmful thought habits, in turn, react on the body, causing physical ailments often with symptoms so real, so violent, and so painful that they imitate diseases produced by actual physical degeneration.

The angina pectoris of the worrier is no less terrifyingly painful than the angina pectoris of the victim whose heart is actually damaged. Even physicians who specialize in heart disorders confess that often they are fooled by these mind-body heart disorders which can simulate a degenerative heart ailment so closely that nothing short of taking the heart out of the body and examining it would reveal the true nature of the illness.

A fatigued, run-down, fear-ridden mind needs physical strengthening, not merely a spilling of its disordered contents. It all traces back to those two indisputable precepts of good health proper nutrition and natural living, two health requisites that are becoming increasingly difficult to follow in the accelerating pace of life in this Early Atomic Age.

The secret of our fathers and grandfathers must be consciously sought by us today. Natural living is difficult under the schedule of twentieth-century living, while proper nutrition is almost impossible through food alone when that food is grown many thousands of miles away in mineral-depleted soils, picked and shipped green, and brought to the table with most of its rich vitamin content sadly dissipated.

To neglect these two rules of good health proper nutrition and natural living is to create a vicious circle, inasmuch as an abused, undernourished, harassed body must necessarily house a mind incapable of optimum thinking and reasoning power.

Correct feeding of the brain tissues makes for healthy thinking. This is axiomatic because the brain, as an organ of the body, is just as susceptible to malnutrition as the eyes, the stomach or the kidneys.

In fact, science has discovered a vitamin and an amino acid that have the power to act directly upon the human brain to increase intelligence. We will talk more about this later.

Therefore, the brain, as the "central power station" of the body, must be kept in top physical condition through natural means so that its mental activities can be controlled, and not allowed to run riot, causing all manner of havoc among the other organs and glands of the body.

A well-nourished mind has every chance to avoid, or to overcome, unhealthy thought habits before they can make irremediable inroads on the body's mechanism. It is true that thought habits of years' and years' duration cannot be changed overnight. Yet, if the brain is a healthy organ, these thought habits can be made to respond, little by little, to proper discipline until the glad day arrives when the physical body is freed of domination by a tense mind.

With our minds able to produce symptoms of diseases that can be cleared up as soon as the mind is strengthened physically and swept clean of its cobweb thinking, and with the ablest of our physicians and surgeons frequently deluded into treating an ailment by drugs and surgery when actually the mind is at fault, it would seem to me that the clearest, sanest course of action before health authorities today is to make the people conscious of the fact that at least half if not all the cure lies within the patient's own mental powers.

In other words, if we build and maintain physically strong, active brain cells, we take out the best health insurance known.

I believe that the health authorities should go even further and warn the people that if they persist in continuing on this mad, hectic, unnatural routine which they have set up as necessary to "civilized" living, then they cannot hope to escape the even madder, more artificial routines which the Atomic Age promises to bring forth.

And the more hectic our existence becomes, the greater will be the price paid in human fatigue a fatigue that will take its toll in more and graver "civilized" diseases, to say nothing of actual mental breakdowns, if more attention is not paid immediately to the brain as a physical organ of the body, needing proper nourishment and good mental hygiene.

"Enjoy yourself; it is later than you think."

Truly, it is later than we think from a mind-body health standpoint. The accumulated worries, fears and violent emotions of the past three decades of increasingly artificial living are giving rise to a bumper crop of physical diseases of purely mental origin.

And the cumulative effect of years of inadequate nutrition is making possible the weakened brain cells that become obsessed with tense emotions. The future in this bewildering Atomic Age will belong to those persons who have schooled themselves in calm mental control and who adhere faithfully to a wise physical regimen.

The person who can retain his mental and physical equilibrium in this New Age will be the person who has learned the treachery of brain and nerve cell fatigue, and who has mastered the secret of how to combat it successfully. Will you be one of these prudent persons?

Chapter 7

The Brain Muscle

Ever since that remote period years ago when prehistoric man first developed enough brain cells to reason, he has been pondering over the solution to two great problems: First, how to develop a sure way to predict the future; and second, how to discover an infallible method of increasing his brain power.

As much as I would delight in doing so, I cannot report any astounding advances in the science of prognostication or clairvoyance. But I am happy to be able to pass on the momentous news about the possibility of increasing brain power! Recent experiments encourage the belief that the brain cells can be so strengthened by certain food elements that they will develop a natural resistance to domination by the type of wrong thought processes which bring on mind-induced illnesses.

As miraculous as the entire idea may seem at first, it now appears reasonably certain that man can do something about increasing his brain capacity through nutrition! In tests on children and teenagers, two food elements have proved their power to raise the intelligence level. This is wonderful news!

If we could raise the intelligence level for thousands and thousands of persons, their mental and emotional troubles could be reduced to an absolute minimum. This would accomplish more lasting good for the mental health of the nation than psychiatry can ever hope to achieve.

Man has always wanted to be more intelligent than he is. He has sought magical ways to give himself mental superiority over his associates; he has swallowed weird brews and dined on gruesome messes all with the one idea of making himself smarter.

Anthropologists report that among savage tribes the brains of astute animals such as the pig, the fox, the ape or the elephant were eagerly sought after as viands sure to increase the intelligence of all who partook of them.

Among cannibalistic tribes, it was almost a sacred rite to serve up to the chief tribesmen the brains of a deceased tribal wizard or medicine man before his burial. Primitive man labored under the impression that the accumulated wisdom and brain-power of one being, either animal or human, could be absorbed by another through consuming the cerebral contents of that body.

As ghoulish as that theory may sound to modern readers, there happens to be one element of truth in it: Greater brain power can arrive via the stomach! Nutritionists have more or less substantiated the half-superstition, half-truth that fish, with its rich supply of phosphorus, is food for the brain.

The only trouble with fish as a brain food is that, in order to change appreciably the capacity of his mental powers, a person would have to consume greater quantities of seafood than his appetite or stomach would tolerate.

The phosphorus in fish is mildly effective in supplying phosphorus for the brain, but not in amounts sufficient to increase greatly the power of the brain cells.

Yet there are two nutritional elements which act directly on the brain. Several all-important experiments recently have substantiated what we nutritionists had begun to realize some years ago: Our brain cells are the sum total of what we do or do not eat!

Science has proved almost conclusively that two separate nutritional elements act directly upon the human brain, thereby increasing its efficiency, thinking power and emotional stability.

These two brain-conditioning food elements are glutamic acid, one of the amino acids which, in turn, make up all food proteins; and thiamin, perhaps known to you as vitamin B-1, and which we have already met in the preceding chapter as the food element necessary to a healthy central nervous system.

The story of the experiments conducted with glutamic acid and thiamin is dramatic enough to capture anyone's imagination. Mental stimulus, to an almost unbelievable degree, was given the subjects of these experiments through simple nutritional substances.

Chapter 8

Glutamic Acid

For our little health drama, let's set the stage first with a nine-year-old girl. She is not a pretty child. Your first impression of her is one of pity rather than admiration. Her dull eyes stare from a vacant, expressionless face.

Little Marie, as we shall call her, is what is known as "stupid." In spite of her nine years, she is hopelessly outclassed by the bright-eyed, active youngsters in her own age group. Marie suffered a serious brain injury during her premature birth.
At the age of five she could only mumble an unintelligible jargon not understood even by her own mother. Although by the time she had reached the age of nine she had learned to form a few understandable words, still she lacked the

mental spark which makes healthy, active children.

Marie would sit all day, like a living soul in a dead body, staring out the window for hours on end without feeling the urge to join in the happy games of the other children.

A long, hopeless life of moronic torpidity stretched before little Marie on the day when she first was taken before the research scientists at Columbia University, along with 43 other mentally retarded children, 11 epileptics, and 14 normal children.

For six months Marie and her fellow patients in the experimental group (ranging in age from sixteen months to seventeen years) were fed pure glutamic acid three times daily. The dose for each child ranged from 6 to 24 grams.

Before the experiment with glutamic acid started, Marie, together with the other patients, was given an intelligence test in which she scored a miserable 69, a rating that marked her as mentally defective. But, at the end of the six-month treatment with glutamic acid, Marie scored 87 (almost normal) in the same type of test.

Even more wonderful than this: Marie became interested in reading a pleasure she had never before been able to enjoy. She learned to bounce a ball with reasonable accuracy.

And when the other little girls gathered on the sidewalk with their jump-ropes, Marie was among them, as eager for her turn as her playmates who had never been handicapped by a subnormal mentality. Glutamic acid has given Marie the promise of a normal life, despite the tragic circumstances surrounding her birth.

Although the case of Marie has been singled out from this group of 44 mentally retarded children selected for this astonishing experiment, the results with the other 43 were equally as promising. In fact, the scientists who conducted the experiment reported that from a medical point of view the most significant cases were those of the defective children, like Marie, whose intelligence was increased to almost normal after only those few months of treatment with glutamic acid.

However, the results obtained with a seventeen-year-old boy in the group, who had a good average intelligence to begin with, were no less remarkable. Before starting the experiment, he scored 107 on the intelligence test, which indicated a normal average mentality.

Yet, after six months of concentrated feedings of glutamic acid, this same boy scored 120 on a similar test, thereby being elevated to the "superior intelligence" class which is only a slight degree below that of "genius." But perhaps the most interesting fact about the entire experiment with these children was the remarkable effect glutamic acid had upon their behavior patterns and personality traits.

Before the experiment, many of the children were disobedient, stubborn, sulky, violently wilful, and belligerent. But the effects of glutamic acid on these same children were marked: they became alert, cooperative, eager to please, good-tempered, and intelligently obedient.

Here you may find the first common sense approach toward curing the juvenile delinquency which is ruining the lives of many of our future citizens. Further, here you may find the answer to the problems that disturbed thinking creates in so many adult minds, wrecking homes, distorting lives and creating a host of psychosomatic illnesses.

The glutamic acid fed to these children during the experiment at Columbia University was administered in pure form either as a powder or in tablets. The pure form of this amino acid is used in research work, since it gives quicker, surer results, primarily owing to the fact that the dose can be accurately measured.

This is not to say that glutamic acid does not occur in foods, for it does, and abundantly so in any protein food. One quart of milk would provide about the minimum daily dose of glutamic acid used in the experiment, whereas four quarts of milk would yield the largest dose given.

One pound of cheddar cheese would contain about the same quantity of glutamic acid, as would one pound of whole wheat or corn bread.

However, if the average child or adult, for that matter were to consume a whole pound of cheese, or four quarts of milk, or an entire loaf of bread per day, it would more than likely upset his dietary balance.

Therefore, the logical way in which to take advantage of glutamic acid for increasing brain power is to use it in pure form as a supplement to a diet containing ample daily portions of lean meats, eggs, natural cheddar cheese (not the process "cheese" foisted onto the public as a "natural" food), milk, peanuts, whole grains, soybeans and other legumes.

With a diet containing the glutamic acid foods as mentioned above, plus glutamic acid in pure form as a safety margin, the same results can be accomplished with both children and adolescents as those reported by Columbia University.

But I must emphasize that rather large amounts of supplementary glutamic acid are needed for the brain cells to derive benefit. This is true because other organs of the body the liver, for instance compete strongly for any glutamic acid contained in the regular diet.

And this demand by the other organs seems to take precedence over the brain's need for glutamic acid. In other words, it is as though Nature decided that since we could go on living without much intelligence, the vital organs should have first call on whatever glutamic acid came into the body, letting the brain wait for the time when enough of this amino acid would be supplied so that every part of the body could have a fair share. Therefore, to assure that enough of this amino acid will be left over for the brain, sufficient glutamic acid must be taken into the body daily so that all organs requiring it will "get theirs" and still leave enough for the brain tissues.

The average person gets slightly less than half an ounce of glutamic acid in his daily diet; and, of course, much less if the diet is seriously deficient in the foods which contain this amino acid. From this it can be realized that glutamic acid as a brain-conditioner can function at maximum efficiency only when provided in the diet in pure form.

How does glutamic acid go about producing this extraordinary effect on tired, dull, underactive minds? When we speak of "intelligence," we are talking about an abstract, intangible power which results very concretely from the number and condition of our brain cells.

In like manner, vision is an abstract ability resulting from a very definite instrument, the eye. To retain the priceless gift of good sight, the physical instrument the eye must be kept in good condition through proper care. In the same way, that intangible power known to us as "intelligence" can be developed and maintained only through proper care of the brain cells.

When talking about "proper care" for any part of the physical body and this includes the brain since it is a vital organ four inviolable rules are presupposed:

- Reasonable precaution to protect the body and its parts from exterior or interior damage by some outside force, such as abuse, overuse or accident.

- Regular rest for the body and its parts to assure needed repairs for tissues damaged by fatigue.

- Efficient elimination to dispose of dead tissue cells and all waste matter, thereby preventing putrefaction and disease within healthy parts.

- Adequate and appropriate nutrition for the tissues composing the body and its different parts.

It is with this fourth and most universally neglected rule of physical health that we are concerned when describing how glutamic acid can increase brain power.

Seriously undernourished brain cells can no more produce mental powers to the fullest degree than a blind eye can see the stars! Atrophied brain cells (atrophied be-cause of cellular starvation) can no more produce the electrical energy demanded for intelligent thinking than atrophied muscles can develop the power needed to lift a book from the table.

67

Brain cells need stimulating food just as the muscles need energy food and the eyes need strengthening food.

Significantly, glutamic acid is the only one of the twenty-three amino acids which is known definitely to be metabolized by the brain tissues.

For a substance to be "metabolized" within the body means that it is "used" by certain parts of the body, thereby becoming altered from its original form, just as the chunk of coal in the stove, after being "used," emerges as smoke, gas and ashes.

Oxygen in the air, for example, is metabolized in the lungs, and then exhaled as carbon dioxide, merely because the blood has taken what it wants of the oxygen in the inhaled air, leaving in its place the waste gas, carbon dioxide, to be expelled.

We have discovered that the brain "uses" glutamic acid, leaving it changed in chemical form, the same as the air which goes into the lungs as oxygen and comes out as carbon dioxide.

This means that this amino acid exerts a direct, beneficial influence upon the brain. In other words, glutamic acid energizes the brain tissues.

This does not mean that glutamic acid increases the actual number of brain cells with which each one of us is endowed. According to all evidence, what glutamic acid really does is to heighten the efficiency of the brain cells we already possess.

This was forcefully illustrated in the case of the seventeen-year-old boy of good average intelligence who soared to the "near genius" class after glutamic acid had raised the efficiency of his brain cells.

Glutamic acid stimulates sluggish brain cells; it prods inactive brain cells into action. Glutamic acid is the ringmaster who keeps the brain performance going at scheduled speed.

Certainly, even this "toning up" of the average brain would add significantly to the intelligence of the world. For, as a famous brain specialist once phrased it: "The average person coasts along, utilizing less than one-third of his normal brain cell capacity."

The way most of us plod along each day, using only one-third of our potential intelligence, can be compared to the man with a powerful eight-cylinder automobile who carelessly allows that super-motor to chug along on two cylinders, wasting completely the potential power of the other six cylinders.

But the brain specialist who accused us of "coasting along" on our mental powers failed to take into account the now evident fact that the other two-thirds of our brain capacity may be idle wholly because it cannot get the proper "fuel" with which to function at top speed.

We have seen that other organs of the body, such as the liver, are the first to receive their share of the scanty amounts of glutamic acid contained in the average diet, leaving little if any for our brain cells.

What if not enough glutamic acid remains for the entire brain? Isn't it logical to suppose, in such an event, that the brain "closes off" a portion of our thinking capacity as we would close off a room in a house to save fuel keeping active only that part for which it can be assured adequate nourishment?

Perhaps the logical way to bring alive that other two-thirds of our unused brainpower is to fuel it up with plenty of glutamic acid. I, for one, have reason to believe that the experiments thus far conducted with glutamic acid have no more than scratched the surface in comparison with what will someday be discovered regarding the heightening effect of glutamic acid on the brain power of the adult mind.

I hope that a growing knowledge of the brain-conditioning powers of glutamic acid will greatly lessen the injudicious use of the drug Benzedrine sulphate which seems currently to be enjoying an ill-deserved vogue among the public, as well as with some medical men.

Used indiscriminately as a stimulant, Benzedrine sulphate can be a very harmful, dangerous drug. You do not need to take my word for this. Here is what the United States Dispensatory has to say about this now popular drug:

The widespread popular use of Benzedrine sulphate to overcome depression, the result of fatigue or alcoholism, is to be greatly deprecated, for three reasons:

- The apparent tendency toward habit formation

- The almost certain rise of blood pressure, and the fact that under some circumstances not understood it may produce dangerous circulatory collapse.

Smith (J.A.M.A., 1939, vol. 113, p. 1022) reports a case of such collapse ending fatally. Certain professional persons, such as writers, attorneys, actors, inventors, artists, musicians, aviators and scientists, who need maximum brain power to carry on their work, despite inadequate rest and indifferent nutrition, have been resorting in recent years to Benzedrine sulphate to give them that greatly desired mental lift.

However, Benzedrine and all other such drug stimulants make their users pay for this lift by exacting from them the toll of an equally violent "drop."

These drugs act directly on the central nervous system, as well as the sympathetic nervous system, whipping up the nerve cells. And, as is true with all artificial over-stimulation, there follow the inevitable let-down and depression.

No synthetic exhilaration conferred upon its user by Benzedrine, or any other drug, can possibly be worth the violence of the reaction which follows the false stimulation of the nervous system.

For those persons who feel as though an added brain stimulus is needed, let me urge that in addition to sane diet, plenty of rest and outdoor exercise they give glutamic acid a chance to do for them naturally what they have been seeking through harmful drugs such as caffeine, nicotine, alcohol or Benzedrine sulphate.

Science has demonstrated convincingly that glutamic acid in sufficient quantities can stimulate the central nervous system (through direct action on the brain cells), thereby relieving fatigue, increasing mental alertness, and alleviating undesirable behavior complexes such as inhibitions, frustrations, anxieties and fears.
All this can be accomplished by glutamic acid without producing those dangerous, depressing after-effects which follow the use of a harmfully stimulating drug.

Chapter 9

Thiamin

Like glutamic acid, thiamin is a food element. It is not a drug. Thiamin occurs naturally in foods containing the vitamin B-complex group, such as whole grains, brewer's yeast, meats, egg yolks, molasses and certain legumes. Thiamin is called the "morale" or "nerve" vitamin for a very good reason. As we have seen in the preceding chapter, it has been recognized for several years that persons seriously lacking in thiamin become depressed, unduly anxious and inexplicably nervous. Severe cases of nervous breakdown have responded unusually well to treatment with thiamin. Hence, thiamin might be said to do for the nerves what vitamin A does for the eyes, and what vitamin C does for the gums.

Cases of chronic fatigue that exhibit violently disturbed mental symptoms respond dramatically to treatment with thiamin.

We have reason to believe that thiamin acts on the nerves in one way through its effect on the brain tissues. Recent experiments with laboratory animals offer good evidence that thiamin, as well as glutamic acid, has a share in keeping the brain healthy and alert.

In these experiments with animals, it was proved that when rats were deprived of all thiamin in their diet, they became only half as intelligent in learning to find their way out of a maze as the rats that received adequate thiamin.

In another laboratory, cats that had been deprived of sufficient thiamin showed signs of impairment of the labyrinthine righting reactions, that is, they were unable to right themselves in mid-air as is normally possible.

From this, the scientists concluded that a thiamin deficiency acts on the synoptic centers of the mid-brain. In still another laboratory, research scientists were working with pigeons. When the birds were fed a diet seriously lacking in thiamin, their brain tissue immediately showed a greatly lowered ability to use oxygen.

And, of course, without plenty of oxygen the brain cells cannot function properly any more than other organs of the body can remain healthy without sufficient oxygen.

Therefore, it would seem that thiamin acts upon the brain by enabling it to make use of the oxygen in the bloodstream. Without sufficient thiamin in the diet, the brain is handicapped through not being able to reach out and make full use of the oxygen that flows in the bloodstream throughout the brain tissues.

A happy comparison would be the pot of coffee set on the stove, awaiting the match to the gas burner before it can be heated. The gas is there in the pipe, and the coffee pot is there ready for the flame. But, without the match, the gas cannot be ignited, and the coffee pot must stay cold. Thiamin seems to be the "match" which enables the brain cells to "burn" the oxygen piped to it in the bloodstream.

An experiment with dramatic results was conducted with thiamin at the Presbyterian Orphans' Home in Lynchburg, Virginia, by scientists from Columbia University. In fact, two identical experiments were undertaken, solely because the first one revealed such startling results that the scientists in charge of the work wanted to be certain beyond all doubt that there was no mistake in the results of the first experiment.

At this orphanage there were about 120 children, an average group of youngsters some bright, some normally intelligent, and some tending toward mental dullness, with I. Q. ratings ranging all the way from 64 (deficient) to 142 (brilliant). Half of the children were given three milligrams of thiamin in tablet form each day, in addition to the regular diet served at the orphanage.

 Because the average diet is assumed to contain only one milligram of thiamin daily, this supplemental amount exceeded normal nutrition by exactly three milligrams a very small increase, according to laboratory standards.

The other group of orphans received no thiamin except that contained in their ordinary diet. However, in order to eliminate what is known as the "imaginative factor," this second group was also given tablets each day the same as the first group, except that the pills taken by the second group were nothing more than "bread pills," containing absolutely no thiamin.

After a period of six weeks, the group of children receiving the supplemental thiamin tablets performed all mental and manual tests with about 40 per cent more efficiency than the second group.

One test which was very popular with the children was performed on a machine that imitated driving an automobile. The child sat behind a real steering wheel at the base of which was a regulation brake pedal.

Before him on a screen, in life-like images, suddenly would appear objects, animals, persons, other automobiles. The "driver" had to make split-second decisions to be executed instantaneously via the brake pedal or the steering wheel, exactly as though he were driving a real car on the highway.

The children who received extra thiamin each day performed far better in this test requiring mental alertness than those children who were left to derive their thiamin requirements from the ordinary diet.

Could it be possible that more thiamin in adult diets would eliminate our ever-increasing number of highway accidents and mounting death tolls?

In addition to this surprising increase in brain power and manual dexterity, the first group of children that had received the extra thiamin showed vastly improved eyesight; they developed a better memory for names and faces; they were better able to memorize written material; they grew taller somewhat more quickly than the second group; their hearing in both ears became keener; and they showed less tendency toward head colds than the second group.

One can readily understand why the scientists who conducted this research desired to repeat the experiment to make sure that there was no "fluke" in these truly miraculous results from so small a supplemental dose of thiamin.

Yet the second experiment revealed nothing more except to re-emphasize the startling results of the first: it proved conclusively that small doses of thiamin, taken in addition to the regular diet, were capable of increasing both mental agility and manual efficiency, plus imparting the other greatly desired physical benefits mentioned above. Therefore, thiamin steps up and takes its rightful place beside glutamic acid as the second of the two natural nutritional elements with the power to heighten mental faculties.

Chapter 10

Brain Power

To date no word has come from the research laboratories about experiments with glutamic acid and thiamin on the adult brain, perhaps mainly because tests with children offer more easily tabulated results. This does not mean, however, that the potential ability of glutamic acid and thiamin to sharpen adult brain power should be ignored.

There is no reason why anyone who reads this chapter cannot do his or her own experimenting with glutamic acid and thiamin. These are two harmless food elements readily available to everyone. Any person who feels mentally tired, depressed, emotionally disturbed, foggy-minded, or upset because of forgetfulness is justified in taking advantage of what is already known about glutamic acid and thiamin as brain and nerve conditioners.

No one can deny that the wonderful news about glutamic acid and thiamin and their beneficial effects on the human brain and nerve cells holds out the bright promise of a happier, healthier, emotionally calmer life for everyone young and old! However, I do not want to give the impression that

I think these two remarkable food elements can make mental wizards of our entire nation. Far from it! And just as well, too, for what we need is not more wizardly intellects, but rather more normal intelligences consistently at work every day.

Nor do I believe that any one of us is as normally intelligent as he or she could be!
That is a pretty broad statement to make, but I do so with the assurance that science backs me up in this assertion.

For many reasons, chiefly nutritional, our average intelligence is known to be sinking gradually to a lower level than need be, despite the "moronizing" influences at work to reduce the average American mind to about a thirteen year old level.

We can and must bring our average national intelligence back to the level where keen thinking and far seeing common sense are the rule rather than the exception among a majority of our people.

We must build emotionally controlled minds that no longer threaten to wreck the physical machine by a host of senseless anxieties and fears. Nutrition scientists must help us overcome the damage which inadequate diets and devitalized foods are causing to the brainpower of our people, both young and old.

A public health law that would require nutritional supplements, such as glutamic acid and thiamin, to be included in the daily diet of every man, woman, boy and girl in America might not be as ridiculous as it seems at first glance.

Science has proved the inestimable value of these two natural food elements in raising the capacity of human brain cells to generate more intelligence. Now all that remains to be done is to try to make glutamic acid and thiamin available to everyone in supplemental form, over and above adequate daily diets which must never be neglected.